Prentice Hall's Exploring Biology Series

GENETIC TESTIMONY

A GUIDE TO
FORENSIC DNA PROFILING

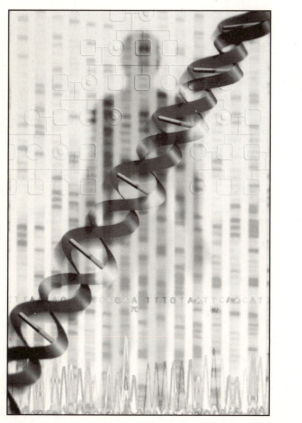

CHARLOTTE A. SPENCER
University of Alberta

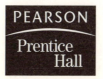

PEARSON

Prentice
Hall

Upper Saddle River, NJ 07458

Editor-in-Chief, Life and Geosciences: Sheri L. Snavely
Executive Editor: Gary Carlson
Project Manager: Crissy Dudonis
Vice President of Production & Manufacturing: David W. Riccardi
Executive Managing Editor: Kathleen Schiaparelli
Assistant Managing Editor: Becca Richter
Production Editor: Elizabeth Klug
Supplement Cover Management/Design: Paul Gourhan
Manufacturing Buyer: Ilene Kahn
Electronic Composition and Formatting: William Johnson
Cover Photo Credit: Stephen Hunt/Getty/Image Bank

© 2004 Pearson Education, Inc.
Pearson Prentice Hall
Pearson Education, Inc.
Upper Saddle River, NJ 07458

Printed in the United States of America

10 9 8 7 6 5 4 3 2 1

ISBN 0-13-142338-X

Pearson Education Ltd., *London*
Pearson Education Australia Pty. Ltd., *Sydney*
Pearson Education Singapore, Pte. Ltd.
Pearson Education North Asia Ltd., *Hong Kong*
Pearson Education Canada, Inc., *Toronto*
Pearson Educación de Mexico, S.A. de C.V.
Pearson Education—Japan, *Tokyo*
Pearson Education Malaysia, Pte. Ltd.
Pearson Education, *Upper Saddle River, New Jersey*

Table of Contents

Preface

Modern forensic DNA profiling is rapidly changing all facets of the criminal justice system. The extreme sensitivity and high levels of discrimination inherent in these methods now make it possible to identify a person who dropped a bloodspot the size of a pinhead or who licked the back of a postage stamp. Crime scene samples that are decades old or ravaged by fire and decay are now yielding profiles that answer questions about identity or guilt.

Forensic DNA profiling names suspects, exonerates the innocent, and identifies the remains of disaster victims. It also challenges traditional forensic methods and pinpoints weaknesses in police techniques and the criminal justice system. As police and governments expand the uses of DNA profiling and compile DNA databanks, questions arise about who should be profiled and how DNA databanks should be regulated.

Over the next decade, it will be increasingly important for all of us to understand the workings of these technologies, why they hold such power, and what shortcomings exist.

In this guide, we explain how current DNA profiling methods work. We also answer questions about the uses of this new technology and how forensic DNA profiling is changing both criminal investigations and the criminal justice system.

The information presented is as current and accurate as possible, and it is derived from scientific literature, the media, and government sources. Because forensic DNA profiling methods are changing rapidly, readers are encouraged to refer to the publication and Internet sources listed in the References and Resources section for the latest developments.

Introduction

"DNA evidence … offers prosecutors important new tools for the identification and apprehension of some of the most violent perpetrators, particularly in cases of sexual assault. At the same time, DNA aids the search for truth by exonerating the innocent. The criminal justice system is not infallible."

Former Attorney General Janet Reno

At 5 P.M. on April 8, 2002, Ray Krone took off his orange jumpsuit, pulled on a T-shirt and a pair of blue jeans, and walked out of the Arizona State Prison into the late afternoon sunshine. After two convictions for a murder he did not commit, after 10 years in prison—three of them on death row—he was a free citizen (Figure 1). "There's tears in my eyes," he said. "Your heart's beating. You can't hardly talk."[1]

Ray Krone and his family never gave up hope that one day the truth would come out—the truth that he did not sexually assault and kill Kim Ancona in 1991. But he had to wait in prison for a decade until new DNA profiling techniques could prove his innocence.

On the morning of December 29, 1991, Kim Ancona, a 36-year-old cocktail waitress, was found naked and stabbed to death in the men's washroom of the Phoenix, Arizona, bar where she worked. There was little forensic evidence at the crime scene. No fingerprints were found and no semen was detected. Blood found at the crime scene matched Kim's blood type, and saliva on her body and clothes was of the most common type. The only useful pieces of physical evidence were bite-marks on Kim's breast and neck. When police learned that Ray Krone had offered to help

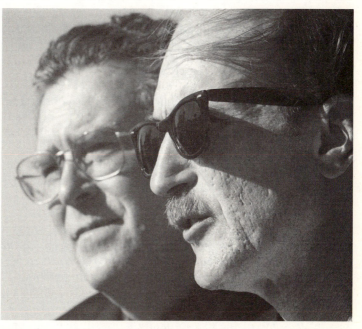

Figure 1
Ray Krone (right) with his lawyer, after release from prison.

SOURCE: AP/World Wide Photos

---

[1]*Arizona Republic*, April 9, 2002, page A1.

Kim close up the bar on the night of the murder, they asked him to make a Styrofoam impression of his teeth for comparison with the crime scene bite-marks. They then arrested him and charged him with first-degree murder, kidnapping, and sexual assault. Krone was assigned an attorney. Prior to his arrest, Krone had no criminal record, had been honorably discharged from the military, and had been a postal worker for seven years.

At his trial, Krone maintained his innocence, saying that he was asleep in bed at the time of the murder. The prosecution's expert witness testified that the bite-marks found on Kim's body matched those on Krone's Styrofoam impression. The prosecution called 19 witnesses, but the defense called only five, including Krone. The jury deliberated for two hours and found him guilty of first-degree murder and kidnapping. The judge sentenced him to death and a consecutive 21-year term of imprisonment.

Ray Krone appealed his sentence and won a new trial in 1996. However, the jury convicted him a second time of first-degree murder and kidnapping, based primarily on the forensic expert's bite-mark testimony. He was sentenced to life in prison rather than death, as the judge admitted having doubts about the identity of the killer.

In 2002, his new defense attorney obtained a court order to test the saliva on Kim Ancona's tank top, using new DNA technology. The results clearly excluded Krone as the source of the saliva, but matched a DNA profile found in the FBI's databank of convicted felons—that of Kenneth Phillips, an inmate serving time for an unrelated sex crime. Although Phillips had lived close to Kim Ancona's bar in 1991, he was not a suspect in her murder.

On April 8, 2002, Ray Krone was released from prison and subsequently exonerated of all convictions. Kenneth Phillips has since been charged with the murder and sexual assault of Kim Ancona.

Krone was the hundredth inmate sentenced to death and subsequently proven innocent and released from prison since 1976, when the U.S. Supreme Court reinstated capital punishment. He was the 12th death row inmate to have his innocence proven by forensic DNA profiling.

A month after his release from prison, Ray Krone stood before a crowd of supporters in his home state of Pennsylvania, vowing to "offer any support I can, anytime, anywhere" to those who seek laws permitting the testing and introduction of DNA evidence to exonerate inmates who are wrongfully convicted.

"I'm thankful to be able to be out here to talk to you all," he said. "DNA made the difference, and I hope that people start realizing the scientific value of DNA and the need for us to update our justice system. And to use this valuable tool, not only to free the innocent, but also to prosecute those that are guilty."[2]

In the last decade, forensic DNA profiling has emerged as a powerful method to identify the guilty and exonerate the innocent. What makes it such a powerful technique? How does DNA profiling work? What are the advantages and drawbacks to the technology, and how is DNA profiling changing the way the criminal justice system functions?

In this guide, we will answer these questions, outlining the basic methods used in forensic DNA profiling and explaining how DNA evidence has the power to convict or exonerate. We will also relate some of the extraordinary stories that have come to light as this new technology expands and transforms criminal justice systems throughout the world.

---

[2]*York Daily Record*, May 8, 2002, page 1A.

Questions About DNA Profiling Methods

WHAT IS THE BIOLOGICAL BASIS FOR FORENSIC DNA PROFILING?

The same DNA is found in virtually all cells in our bodies

Each of us is made up of hundreds of billions of cells, each one of which is derived by cell division from a single fertilized egg. Our cells contain two main compartments—the cytoplasm and the nucleus (Figure 2). An exception is the red blood cell, which contains no nucleus. Within the nucleus are the chromosomes—threadlike structures that carry the genetic material. Human cells contain 23 pairs of chromosomes, one of each pair inherited from the mother via the egg cell and one of each pair inherited from the father via the sperm cell. Males inherit a Y chromosome from the father's sperm, whereas females inherit an X chromosome. Therefore, each person is either an XY male or an XX female (Figure 3).

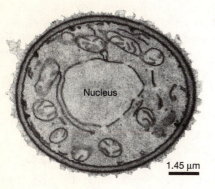

Nucleus

1.45 µm

Figure 2
Microscopic view of a single cell. Cells are comprised of a nucleus which contains the chromosomes, and the cytoplasm which contains structures called mitochondria. Both mitochondria and nuclear chromosomes contain DNA.

SOURCE: Scott Freeman, *Biological Sciences*, Prentice Hall

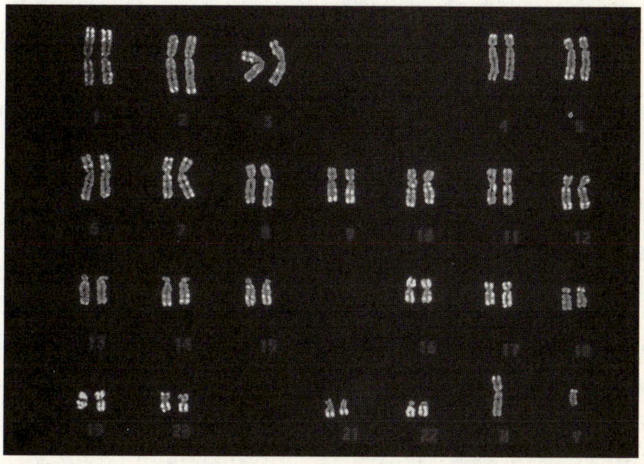

Figure 3
Human chromosomes, seen at high magnification. The nucleus of each human cell contains 23 pairs of chromosomes—22 autosomal chromosomes and one pair of sex chromosomes. This set of chromosomes was derived from a male (XY).

SOURCE: William S. Klug and Michael R. Cummings, *Concepts of Genetics*, Prentice Hall

Genetic information is contained within the base pair sequence of DNA

Each chromosome is made up of a single linear molecule of DNA (deoxyribonucleic acid). Each DNA molecule is comprised of two strands coiled around each other in a double helix. Each single strand is made up of a repetitive sugar-phosphate backbone to which are linked four *bases*, arranged in various orders (Figure 4). The bases are known as A, T, C, and G (abbreviations for adenine, thymine, cytosine, and guanine). These chemical bases pair with each other by hydrogen bonding and hold the two strands of the double helix together. The T base always pairs with A, and the G base always pairs with C. The base pairs on each DNA molecule are arranged in a specific order, like a four-letter Morse code. This is known as the *DNA sequence*. Because A always pairs with T, and G always pairs with C, the DNA sequences on each strand are *complementary* to each other. There are about 6 billion base pairs of DNA in a human cell. The entire complement of DNA in a cell's nucleus is known as the *genome*.

A *gene* is a portion of DNA of about 1,000 to 100,000 base pairs in length. There are approximately 30,000 genes in the entire human genome. Each gene occupies a specific region on a specific chromosome. Specific regions of a chromosome, whether occupied by genes or not, are known as *loci*. Each is a *locus*. The cell reads the linear sequence of base pairs within a gene and converts that information into the linear sequence of amino acids in a particular protein. In this way, each gene specifies the synthesis of one specific protein.

DNA sequences differ between individuals

Although humans are fundamentally similar, enough genetic difference exists between individuals to make each of us detectably unique. Most of our DNA sequences are identical, but approximately one base pair in 1,000 differs between individuals. As there are 6 billion base pairs in the human genome, this means that about 6 million base pairs differ between individuals. This small amount of genetic diversity accounts for slight differences in the proteins found in cells and hence the range of physical differences seen in humans. These DNA sequence differences are also the basis for forensic DNA profiling. If we could compare the complete DNA sequences from two people, we could be certain that the DNA came from two distinct individuals.

Alternative forms of a gene or locus, due to the presence of DNA sequence differences, are known as *alleles*. If a person's cells contain the same allele of a gene on each of a chromosome pair (one from the mother and one from the father), that person is said to be *homozygous* for that gene. If the person's cells contain two different alleles of the gene, they are said to be *heterozygous* for that gene. For example, if you inherit the *A* allele of Gene A and the *b* allele of Gene B from your mother, and the *a* allele of Gene A and the *b* allele of Gene B from your father, you are an *Aa* heterozygote for Gene A and a *bb* homozygote for Gene B. Another way this is expressed is that your *genotype* is *Aa/bb*.

When egg and sperm cells develop, the chromosome pairs separate, and each member of a chromosome pair is distributed randomly to the egg or sperm. This independent segregation of chromosomes, combined with recombination events during egg and sperm development, creates an enormous variety of genetic allele combinations in eggs and sperm. This means that even siblings are genetically different, although less different than two people chosen at random from a population. The only individuals with an identical genetic makeup are identical twins, who develop from a single fertilized egg. In a population, there are usually numerous different alleles for any gene or locus. This is known as gene *polymorphism*.

NUCLEOTIDES ARE THE BUILDING BLOCKS OF DNA

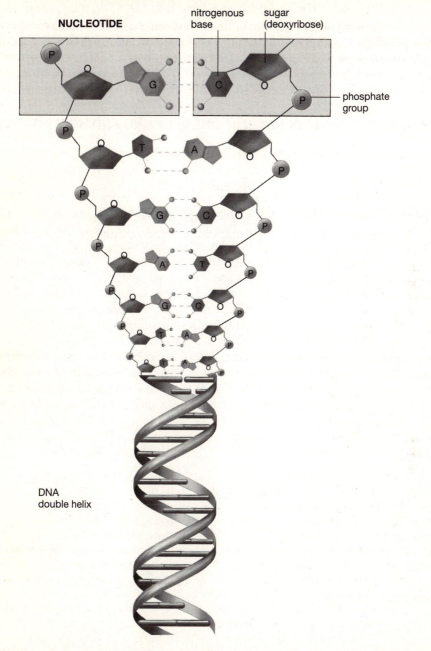

Figure 4

Diagram of DNA molecule, showing double helix, sugar-phosphate backbone and bases A, T, G, and C. Hydrogen bonds between the bases of the two single strands hold the double helix together. These bonds can be broken by heat, chemicals or enzymes. The DNA sequence of this molecule would be **G T G A G T T** on one strand, and **C A C T C A A** on the complementary strand.

SOURCE: David Krogh, *Biology: A Guide to the Natural World*, Prentice Hall

Surprisingly, coding regions of genes make up only about 5% of the human genome. The remaining 95% of human DNA is sometimes called "junk DNA," as it is unclear what functions are performed by much of this material. These noncoding regions are particularly useful for forensic DNA analysis, as they are rich in tandomly repeated DNA sequences. These repeats can vary from two base units (e.g., AT) repeated from two to dozens of times (ATAT to ATATATATAT etc.), up to 80 base units repeated from two to dozens of times. These repeat regions are the basis for many of the DNA profiling methods used in forensics.

WHAT METHODS ARE USED IN FORENSIC DNA PROFILING AND HOW DO THEY WORK?

Variable number of tandem repeat (VNTR) methods

Background

The first use of DNA profiling in a criminal investigation occurred in 1986 in the United Kingdom, and it involved the analysis of large repeat areas of DNA called variable number of tandem repeat (VNTR) regions (see box: The Colin Pitchfork Story). In 1988, the Federal Bureau of Investigation (FBI) and U.S. commercial laboratories began using VNTR DNA profile methods.

The VNTRs contain DNA sequence units eight to 80 base pairs long repeated consecutively along the chromosome. The number of tandem repeats in each VNTR locus differs from person to person. A VNTR may contain anywhere from a thousand to several thousand base pairs of DNA. Each of these tandem repeat lengths is considered to be an allele.

One of the reasons that VNTRs are useful for DNA profiling is the large number of alleles (30 or more) at each VNTR locus that are present in a population. The large number of alleles means that the number of possible genotypes is immense. For example, if there are 20 alleles at VNTR locus A (A1, A2, A3, etc.), the total number of possible genotypes for locus A would be 210. If one analyzed a person's DNA at four different VNTR loci, and each VNTR locus had 20 possible alleles, the number of possible genotypes in this four locus profile would be 210^4 (about 2 billion).

The Colin Pitchfork Story

Between 1983 and 1986, police were unable to solve two murders in the village of Narborough in Leicestershire, England. Two 15-year-old schoolgirls, Lynda Mann and Dawn Ashworth, had been raped, strangled, and thrown into the bushes next to secluded pathways near the town. The perpetrator left no clues at the crime scene except for his semen. Initially, police focused their investigation on a 17-year-old mentally retarded kitchen porter from a nearby mental hospital, as he had a previous history of sexual offences. When questioned, the porter made a full confession to the murder of Dawn Ashworth. Police accepted his confession, but they were interested to know whether the porter might also be responsible for Lynda Mann's death.

Police asked Dr. Alec Jeffreys of the University of Leicester to help them identify the perpetrator of the Mann murder. Dr. Jeffreys had been studying variable number of tandem repeat (VNTR) regions in human populations and had developed methods for measuring the sizes of VNTR loci. Police provided Dr. Jeffreys with semen samples from the girls' bodies, as well as a blood sample from the porter. Dr. Jeffreys' VNTR analysis clearly showed that the DNA profiles of semen from both crime scenes matched, suggesting that the same person had committed the rapes. However, neither DNA profile matched that of the porter. The porter had become the first person in history to be exonerated by DNA profiling.

(continued)

Police now turned their attention to the entire male population of Narborough and surrounding villages. They requested that every adult male in the area provide them with a blood sample to compare with those from the crime scenes. More than 4,000 men provided samples. One man who did not provide a sample was a local bakery worker, Colin Pitchfork. To avoid providing the sample, Pitchfork paid a co-worker, Ian Kelly, to give a sample on his behalf, using a forged passport as identification. The plan would have gone undetected were it not for a conversation overheard at a local pub. Bakery workers were heard discussing the fact that Kelly had given Pitchfork's sample, and one of the pub's patrons reported the conversation to police. Pitchfork was arrested and forced to provide a blood sample. The DNA profile from his blood matched the DNA profile from the semen samples at the crime scene. Pitchfork confessed to the murders, pleaded guilty, and was sentenced to life in prison.

Method for VNTR Profiling

A VNTR DNA profile is created by measuring the lengths of a number of different VNTR loci in a person's DNA. Originally, this method of generating a VNTR profile was called *DNA fingerprinting*. This terminology has now been replaced by *DNA profiling* to differentiate it from classic dermal ridge pattern fingerprinting methods.

The method entails the following (Figure 5):

1. DNA is extracted from the sample using a series of chemical treatments.

2. The DNA is cut into millions of small pieces using a *restriction enzyme*, which recognizes specific sequences in the DNA and makes double-stranded cuts through the DNA at those positions. For example, the restriction enzyme *Hae*III recognizes the DNA sequence GGCC. It then cuts the DNA between the G and C. For example (showing a short region of double-stranded DNA):

   ---ATCGTTAGGCCTCAAG--- → ---ATCGTTAGG--- ---CCTCAAG---
   ---TAGCAATCCGGAGTTC---   ---TAGCAATCC--- ---GGAGTTC---

   Restriction enzymes are chosen that do not cut within the VNTR locus, but cut the DNA on either side of it. Because the recognition sequences for restriction enzymes occur throughout the DNA molecule, but at various distances from each other, the DNA is cut into pieces that vary in length from a few base pairs to thousands of base pairs.

3. The DNA sample is placed in a well at the end of a slab of jelly-like material (called a *gel*) and an electrical charge is passed through the gel. Smaller-sized DNA fragments migrate more quickly through the gel than do larger fragments. This process is called *gel electrophoresis*. The distance that a particular fragment travels down the gel depends upon its size.

4. Because the gel is fragile and difficult to handle, the DNA in the gel is transferred onto a nylon membrane. The DNA is treated with alkali, so that the two strands of the double helix denature (come apart), exposing the bases.

5. Up until now, the DNA fragments are not detectable on either the gel or on the membrane. In order to detect the VNTR fragments, the membrane bearing the DNA fragments is incubated in a solution containing a *probe*. The probe consists of single-stranded DNA, which is complementary in its DNA sequence to the VNTR region that is of interest. The probe also contains a tag—either radioactivity or a chemical

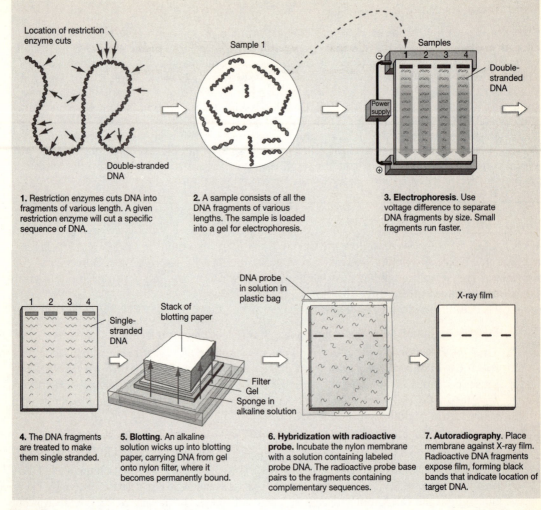

Figure 5
Method of creating a VNTR profile

SOURCE: Scott Freeman, *Biological Science*, Prentice Hall

that emits light. The probe *hybridizes* (binds) to any piece of DNA on the membrane that bears the complementary DNA sequence (following the A-T, G-C base-pairing rules).

6. The excess probe that does not hybridize to the VNTR DNA fragments is washed off.

7. The membrane with its hybridized probe is exposed to X-ray film. Positions on the membrane that contain the probe (and hence the VNTR of interest) create an image on the film and show up as bands. The resulting photographic image is known as an *autoradiograph*. The position of the bands within the lane of DNA fragments, when compared to standard size markers in adjacent lanes, indicates the size of the fragment in each band. A typical VNTR analysis is shown in Figure 6, and an example of a VNTR autoradiograph is shown in Figure 7.

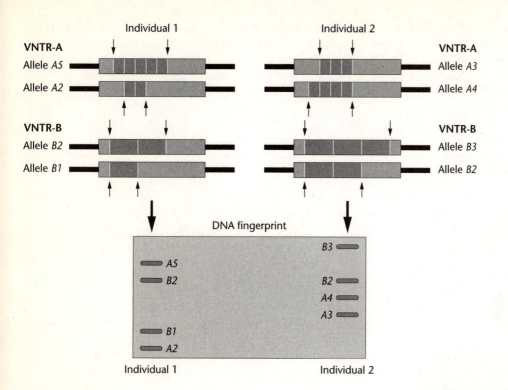

Individual 1

VNTR-A
Allele *A5*
Allele *A2*

VNTR-B
Allele *B2*
Allele *B1*

Individual 2

VNTR-A
Allele *A3*
Allele *A4*

VNTR-B
Allele *B3*
Allele *B2*

DNA fingerprint

A5
B2

B1
A2

B3

B2
A4
A3

Individual 1

Individual 2

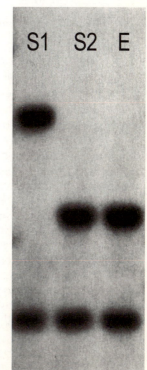

S1   S2   E

▲ **Figure 6**
Two VNTR loci in two individuals and their analysis by VNTR profiling.
Arrows indicate the sites of cutting by restriction enzymes. The DNA
fragments are separated by gel electrophoresis and detected as bands
after probing the membrane with a labelled probe and exposing the
membrane to X-ray film. Because the sizes of the VNTR fragments differ
between individuals, the bands on the autoradiograph appear at different
positions. In these profiles, one band (the B2 allele band) is shared by the
two individuals.

SOURCE: William S. Klug and Michael R. Cummings, *Concepts of
Genetics*, Prentice Hall

▶ **Figure 7**
An example of a VNTR autoradiograph. The DNA profile of Suspect 2
(S2) matches that of the crime scene evidence (E). Suspect 1 (S1) is
excluded as the source of the crime scene evidence. Both suspects share
one allele at this VNTR locus.

SOURCE: William S. Klug and Michael R. Cummings, *Concepts of
Genetics*, Prentice Hall

Usually, the DNA samples to be compared are placed in adjacent lanes on the same gel. If the two VNTR bands from one DNA sample run at different positions on the gel from the two VNTR bands from another DNA sample, they are considered a nonmatch, and the two samples must have come from different people. However, if the two samples show the same-sized VNTR bands, the profiles are considered a match. A match means that either the two DNA samples

---

Polymerase Chain Reaction

The polymerase chain reaction (PCR) is a method for generating multiple copies of specific regions of DNA. The PCR technique is based on the principles of DNA base pairing and DNA replication, and it consists of four steps:

1. DNA is extracted from the sample. This is the template DNA. It is mixed with:

   - A solution of four dNTPs (building blocks of the DNA molecule, containing a sugar, phosphate, and one of the bases A, T, G, or C).
   - A heat-resistant DNA polymerase enzyme called Taq polymerase.
   - A solution containing millions of copies of specific PCR primers. The PCR primers are very short (about 20 bases long) single-stranded DNA molecules that have been synthesized in the laboratory and have defined DNA sequences. The primer sequences are chosen to flank the region that is to be amplified.

2. The reaction mixture is heated to 95°C for 5 minutes, which causes the two strands of the DNA double helix to denature, exposing the bases.

3. The temperature is lowered to between 50° and 70°C for several minutes. The primers hybridize to their complementary base pair sequences present in the template DNA.

4. Taq polymerase extends the primers by adding dNTPs to the 3′ ends of the primers, filling in the gaps between the primers and creating double-stranded DNA in the region between the primers.

Steps two to four are repeated 20 to 30 times. At each cycle, the number of double-stranded DNA molecules doubles. Two single strands of the target DNA yield two double-stranded copies. The two copies now act as templates for the creation of four copies, and so on, up to a million-fold increase in the amount of DNA of the target sequence. The PCR reaction is carried out in a single test tube, and the entire process is automated in machines called *thermocyclers*.

Because the PCR method selectively amplifies a specific short region of a DNA molecule, the template DNA for the first PCR cycle can be impure, present in minuscule amounts (theoretically one molecule), and can be partially degraded, as long as one DNA molecule in the sample has an intact amplification region. These features make PCR particularly useful for forensic DNA analysis, which can be performed on single hairs, a small number of cells in saliva on the back of a postage stamp, or decayed samples from old crime scenes.

Once the relevant regions of DNA have been amplified by PCR, they can be analyzed using a number of different methods, such as STR, SNP, mtDNA, and Y chromosome DNA profiling—as described in this guide.

(continued)

The great sensitivity and power of PCR—amplifying a single copy of a DNA molecule into millions of copies—also creates a potential problem. Any contamination of the DNA sample with DNA from another source could potentially result in amplification of the wrong DNA, or amplification of a mixture of two types. This is a particular problem when trace amounts of material must be amplified for forensic DNA profiling. If the contaminating DNA is present in small amounts compared with the primary DNA, the PCR products from the contaminant will be present in lower concentrations than will those from the primary DNA. However, if only a few cells of both primary and contaminant samples are present, a mixed DNA profile or an incorrect one may be generated. These limitations must be kept in mind when analyzing PCR-based DNA profiles.

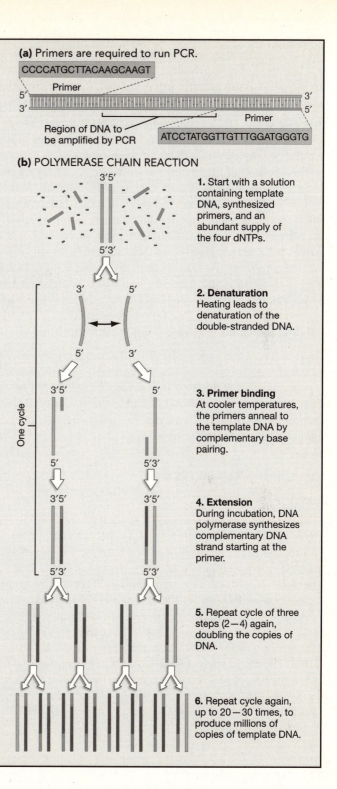

(a) Primers are required to run PCR.

CCCCATGCTTACAAGCAAGT

Primer

5′   3′
3′   5′

Region of DNA to be amplified by PCR

Primer

ATCCTATGGTTGTTTGGATGGGTG

(b) POLYMERASE CHAIN REACTION

3′5′
5′3′

1. Start with a solution containing template DNA, synthesized primers, and an abundant supply of the four dNTPs.

3′   5′
5′   3′

2. Denaturation
Heating leads to denaturation of the double-stranded DNA.

One cycle

3′5′   5′

3. Primer binding
At cooler temperatures, the primers anneal to the template DNA by complementary base pairing.

5′   5′3′

3′5′   3′5′

4. Extension
During incubation, DNA polymerase synthesizes complementary DNA strand starting at the primer.

5′3′   5′3′

5. Repeat cycle of three steps (2—4) again, doubling the copies of DNA.

6. Repeat cycle again, up to 20—30 times, to produce millions of copies of template DNA.

Steps in the polymerase chain reaction technique.
SOURCE: Scott Freeman, *Biological Science*, Prenctice Hall

came from the same person, or they came from two different people who share the same geno-type by chance. Probability calculations can estimate the likelihood of such a random match at any locus or a combination of loci.

After an autoradiograph has been created from the membrane, the membrane is stripped of its probe by washing at high temperature. The membrane is then treated with a different probe that will hybridize to the DNA from a different VNTR locus. Usually, at least five or six different VNTR loci are analyzed to create a DNA profile. Each cycle of probing, film exposure and stripping takes several days or weeks, meaning that it requires weeks or months to generate a VNTR DNA profile.

This method of measuring variable sizes of DNA fragments that have been cut by restriction enzymes is sometimes known as *restriction fragment length polymorphism (RFLP)* analysis.

The VNTR profiling has several limitations. Relatively large amounts of DNA are necessary to detect the presence of fragments on a gel or membrane—about the amount of DNA from a blood stain the size of a quarter. The DNA must be in good condition (not degraded) in order to create intact VNTR fragments of up to thousands of base pairs in length. In addition, the procedure is slow, taking up to several weeks to analyze several VNTR loci. First used from 1985 to the mid-1990s, VNTR profiling is still used in some cases; however, it has been almost completely replaced by newer methods based on PCR technology, which is described next.

Polymerase chain reaction (PCR)–based methods

To circumvent the limitations of VNTR profiling, forensic scientists have developed a number of new techniques based on the use of PCR, a method for amplifying small quantities of specific regions of DNA prior to analysis (see box: Polymerase Chain Reaction). The PCR method is capable of amplifying DNA in a single cell, and it typically requires about 50-fold less DNA than that required for VNTR analysis. The following is a brief summary of the current DNA profiling methods based on PCR technology.

Short Tandem Repeats (STRs)

Background

Analysis of STRs has essentially replaced VNTR analysis as the method of choice for forensic DNA profiling. Like VNTRs, STRs are regions within a person's DNA that contain specific DNA sequences tandomly repeated a number of times. However, STRs consist of smaller repeat units (two to seven base pairs long) repeated fewer times (seven to 40 repeats per STR region). The short lengths of STR regions allow them to be amplified using the PCR technique, which cannot efficiently amplify the longer VNTR regions.

Although hundreds of STR loci are contained within a person's genome, only a subset of these is used for DNA profiling. At present, the FBI specifies 13 STR loci as a core set to be used in forensic analysis. The core STR loci are listed in Table 1. For example, one STR locus (D8S1179) has 10 alleles (10 different repeat lengths) and has a four base pair repeat unit (TCTA). When all 13 core STR loci are used to generate a DNA profile, the probability that two randomly chosen profiles will match is approximately one in 6×10^{14} (one in 600 trillion) in a Caucasian American population or one in 9×10^{14} (one in 900 trillion) in an African American population.

Locus	Repeat	# Alleles	Population Match Probabilities	
			Caucasian American	African American
CSF1PO	AGAT	11	0.112	0.081
TPOX	AATG	7	0.195	0.090
TH01	AATG	7	0.081	0.109
vWA	TCTA	10	0.062	0.063
D16S539	GATA	8	0.089	0.070
D7S820	GATA	11	0.065	0.080
D13S317	TATC	8	0.085	0.136
D5S818	AGAT	10	0.158	0.112
FGA	TTTC	19	0.036	0.033
D3S1358	TCTA	10	0.075	0.094
D8S1179	TCTA	10	0.067	0.082
D18S51	AGAA	15	0.028	0.029
D21S11	TCTA	20	0.039	0.034
Product			1.738×10^{-15}	1.092×10^{-15}
One in			5.753×10^{14}	9.161×10^{14}

Table 1 Characteristics of the FBI's 13 Core STR Loci

Source: *The Future of Forensic DNA Testing: Predictions of the Research and Development Working Group*, by the National Institute of Justice, November 2000.

Method for STR Profiling

1. DNA is extracted from the sample.
2. The DNA undergoes PCR amplification of the selected STR locus.
3. The sizes of the amplified fragments are measured.

After PCR amplification, the DNA sample will contain a small quantity of the original DNA (the template for the PCR reaction) and a large quantity of amplified DNA of the locus selected for amplification. Because each person has two copies of each STR locus (one on the maternal chromosome, one on the paternal chromosome), there will usually be two STR amplification products of slightly different sizes present in the reaction. At this point, the two products are separated as to size, by one of several methods.

First, the amplified fragments may be analyzed by slab gel electrophoresis—the same method used to analyze VNTR fragments (Figure 5). Following gel electrophoresis, the gel is stained with silver so as to visualize the two amplified STR bands. By comparing the STR bands to the standard DNA size markers on the gel, the size of each band can be computed.

A second method requires that the primers in the PCR reaction bear fluorescent tags. When the primers become incorporated into the amplified DNA fragments, they make those fragments fluorescent. After the PCR amplification step, the amplified DNA fragments are separated by a form of gel electrophoresis called *capillary electrophoresis*. This method uses fine-bore glass capillaries filled with gel material similar to that used in slab gel electrophoresis. The DNA sample is placed at the top of the capillary tube and an electric current is passed through the gel in the capillary. The DNA fragments are separated as to size as they pass down the capillary toward the positive electrode. A laser detector at the bottom of the tube detects fluorescent DNA as it passes the end of the capillary. The data are collected and analyzed by software that calculates the DNA fragment sizes as well as the relative amount of DNA in each band. Data are visualized as graphs showing the position and size of the DNA fragments. Capillary electrophoresis is faster than slab gel electrophoresis, requires less DNA, and is amenable to automation. Automated capillary gel instruments can analyze up to 96 samples over a period of a few hours. An example of an STR DNA profile using this method is shown in Figure 8.

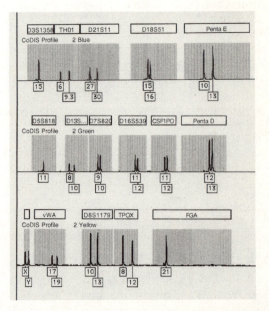

Figure 8
An STR profile, created using the PowerPlex® Kit (Promega Corp.)
This kit amplifies all 13 core STR loci, as well as two extra loci (Penta E and D) and a locus (Amelogenin) that indicates the presence of either an X or a Y chromosome in the DNA sample. Most loci in this profile are heterozygous; however, three loci (D3S1358, D5S818 and FGA) appear to be homozygous. Primers in this reaction were labelled with blue, green or yellow fluorescent dyes, allowing simultaneous amplification of all 16 loci and simultaneous capillary electrophoresis of all loci. The numbers in boxes below each peak indicate the allele (15 repeats, 6 repeats, etc).

SOURCE: H. Edward Grothan

Forensic DNA Databases

The United States, Canada, Australia, China, the United Kingdom and many European countries have established national forensic DNA databases. The first of these databases containing STR profiles was created in the United Kingdom in 1995. In the United Kingdom, all suspects and arrestees are compelled to submit samples for DNA testing. The U.K. database now consists of over 1.5 million DNA profiles and will contain 3 million profiles by 2004. Government figures indicate that about 1,600 DNA matches are obtained each week by searching the database. These either link a suspect to a crime scene or reveal links between different crime scenes.

In 1998, the FBI established a national DNA database, called the Combined DNA Index System (CODIS). All 50 states have laws requiring convicted offenders of certain crimes to submit DNA samples for profiling. At present, all but three states (Hawaii, Rhode Island, and Mississippi) submit these profiles to CODIS. States vary considerably in the types of crimes that qualify for database entry. Some states collect DNA samples from all arrested people, but others collect samples only from offenders convicted of specific violent crimes such as rape and murder.

The CODIS system contains two main criminal DNA databases—the Convicted Offender database and the Forensic Evidence database—as well as one missing persons index. In addition, CODIS contains computer software that allows investigators to search for matches within and across the DNA profile databases, as well as STR allele frequency data from major population groups. The Convicted Offender database contains DNA profiles of individuals convicted of certain violent crimes. The Forensic Evidence database contains DNA profiles from biological evidence samples collected from crime scenes, such as semen, saliva, or bloodstains. The missing persons database contains mtDNA and STR DNA profiles from remains such as bones, teeth, or hair. It also contains DNA profiles from relatives of missing persons, so that comparisons can be made between known and unknown samples.

The FBI has chosen 13 core STR loci as standards for CODIS profiles (Table 1). All 13 loci are used by Canada's Royal Canadian Mounted Police (RCMP) and eight core STR loci are used in the U.K. database, which could facilitate international cross-referencing of DNA profiles.

The DNA profile databases have helped investigations into murders, rapes, burglaries, and even forgeries. These databases are particularly useful in solving *cold cases*—unsolved cases in which there is no suspect. In Virginia, 178 cold hits were obtained in 2000 and about 300 in 2001. By May 2002, CODIS had contributed to 5,000 forensic investigations and had produced over 4,000 DNA profile matches.

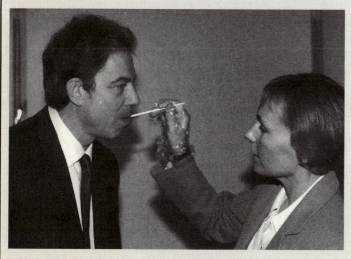

Prime Minister Tony Blair, supporting U.K. DNA legislation by donating a mouth swab for DNA profiling and entry into Britain's national DNA database.

SOURCE: AP/World Wide Photos

In all STR profiling methods, the genotype of the individual is expressed as the allele sizes of the STR fragments. For example, a DNA profile may show alleles of 11 and 12 repeats at the D5S818 locus (expressed as D5S818 11,12) and alleles of eight and nine repeats at the TPOX locus (expressed as TPOX 8,9).

Commercial kits are now available for generating STR-based DNA profiles. In some cases, these kits amplify all 13 core STR loci (as well as other loci) simultaneously in a single reaction, a feature that speeds the analysis and preserves limited amounts of forensic evidence. This type of DNA profiling is termed *multiplexing*.

After a DNA profile is generated, it is compared to another profile from another person or from a crime scene sample. Also, DNA profiles can be compared with profiles stored in national or regional DNA databanks (see box: Forensic DNA Databases).

Single Nucleotide Polymorphisms (SNPs)

A new and emerging method of DNA profiling involves analysis of single nucleotide polymorphisms (SNPs). The SNPs are differences in the DNA sequence at single positions in the genome. An SNP may be due to a single base pair change or to a small insertion or deletion at that position. An example of a single base pair SNP is shown in Figure 9.

Single nucleotide polymorphisms are present about once every 1,000 bases throughout the entire genome, making the number of potential profiling loci enormous (about 6 million). Most SNPs have only two alleles; hence, analysis of a single SNP is not very discriminating for identification purposes. However, when combined with analysis of a large number of other SNP loci, SNP profiling can be as informative as STR or VNTR profiling. At present, SNP loci are being catalogued and characterized for future DNA profiling purposes.

In order to detect SNPs, the DNA is first amplified by PCR. The amplified DNA is then subjected to DNA sequencing. As DNA sequencing is fairly cumbersome, alternate methods for detecting single base pair differences in amplified DNA are currently being developed.

One of the early applications of SNP analysis was known as HLA-DQA1 and Polymarker profiling. In this method, six SNP loci are PCR-amplified and hybridized to filters that contain probe DNA that is specific for each polymorphism. Hybridization is detected by staining. Although simple and accurate, the discriminating power of this method is only about one in 4,000. The method has now been replaced by standard STR analysis.

There are several major advantages to SNP DNA profiling. The human genome contains vast numbers of these loci, their analysis may become automated in the future, and the regions of interest are so small that highly degraded DNA samples are still amenable to PCR amplification and SNP detection. Currently, SNP profiling is being used to identify the remains of victims of the September 11, 2001, terrorist attacks on the World Trade Center in New York (see box: DNA Profiling Identifies September 11 Victims).

5'-----A T C C G A G C T T C A A-----3'
3'-----T A G G C T C G A A G T T-----5'

↓

5'-----A T C C G A G C C T C A A-----3'
3'-----T A G G C T C G G A G T T-----5'

Figure 9
Example of a Single Nucleotide Polymorphism (SNP) creating a single base pair change in a short region of a double-stranded DNA molecule.

DNA Profiling Identifies September 11 Victims

Identifying the remains of victims from the September 11, 2001, terrorist attacks on the World Trade Center in New York has been the largest and most difficult forensic DNA investigation in American history.

By the end of 2002, the official death toll stood at 2,795. About 1.6 million tons of debris has been removed from the site, as well as 293 whole bodies and about 20,000 pieces of bone and tissue—some pieces as small as a fingertip. The trauma of the collapsing skyscrapers pulverized most of the victims' bodies to dust, and much of the remaining fragments were damaged by fire, water, and bacterial degradation.

Bodies and body parts were brought to the Medical Examiner's Office in New York City, where they were stored in 16 refrigerated trailers. From there, they were examined by pathologists, fingerprint experts, and forensic dentists. The initial identifications were made using traditional forensic identification methods, such as fingerprinting and dental records. Only 10 of the victims could be identified visually. In order to identify the partial remains, authorities turned to DNA profiling. The profiling was carried out by the N.Y. Medical Examiner's Office, which assembled the data, and by private DNA analysis laboratories in Utah, Texas, Maryland, and Virginia. In order to match DNA profiles to victims, laboratories collected personal items from the victims' homes—about 7,000 razor blades, combs, toothbrushes, and other items, as well as about 7,000 cheek swabs from the victims' relatives.

The method of choice for the initial DNA profiling was STR (short tandem repeat) analysis—profiling the 13 core STR loci and comparing the profiles with those generated from DNA extracted from the victim's personal property. Half the tissue and bone samples yielded sufficient STR profiles to identify the remains. However, the other half either provided no STR DNA profile or only a partial one.

By September 2002, about half of the World Trade Center victims had been identified. To complete the identification of remains, DNA laboratories are turning to more sensitive profiling methods—mtDNA and SNP (single nucleotide polymorphism) analysis. These profiling methods are capable of generating DNA profiles from highly degraded DNA, even as little as 60 base pairs of intact DNA per locus. The hope is that samples that did not generate a usable STR profile will give sufficient mtDNA or SNP profiles to identify the victim. New mtDNA and SNP profile technologies and new database analysis methods are being developed specifically to deal with the volume and condition of material from the World Trade Center attacks. The new technologies will undoubtedly have an impact on forensic DNA profiling in the future.

The goal is to complete identification of all victims by the middle of 2003.

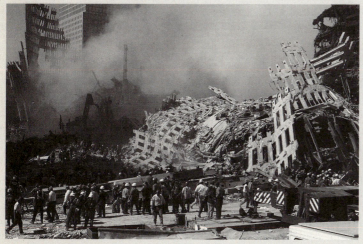

Remains of the World Trade Center, New York, after the September 11 terrorist attacks.

SOURCE: REUTERS/CORBIS BETTMANN

Mitochondrial DNA (mtDNA)

Analysis of mtDNA is a recent addition to the repertoire of forensic DNA profiling. Mitochondria are organelles present in thousands of copies within the cytoplasm of cells, and they are responsible for generating energy via oxidative respiration (Figure 2).

Mitochondria contain their own small (approximately 16,000 base pairs) circular DNA genomes, and they replicate independently of the cell's nuclear chromosomes. When a cell divides, the mitochondria are distributed to the two new daughter cells. Human egg cells contain mitochondria in their cytoplasm and pass these mitochondria on to the zygote. However, sperm cells contain few mitochondria and do not pass these to the zygote on fertilization. Hence, off-spring contain only maternally derived mitochondria. Because of these features, all mtDNA is identical in each cell of the body, and is passed from grandmother to mother to child.

The DNA profiles of mtDNA are generated by PCR amplification of regions of mtDNA that exhibit DNA sequence polymorphisms within populations. Amplification is followed by deter-mination of the DNA sequence in that region. The DNA sequence is then compared with that from a reference sample to determine a match or nonmatch.

Although direct sequencing of mtDNA is still relatively slow and expensive, technical advances may soon make it a standard procedure in forensic science. Databases of mtDNA poly-morphisms and allele frequencies are being compiled.

There are several advantages to mtDNA profiling. Because mtDNA is present in thousands of copies per cell, extremely small amounts of biological material can often be analyzed successfully. Also, severely degraded material such as charred remains and old bones can sometimes be analyzed, even when chromosomal DNA is too severely degraded to yield STR profiles. In addition, mtDNA can be analyzed in samples such as hair shafts, which contain no nuclear DNA. The DNA profiling of mtDNA has been used to identify victims of disasters, assassinations, and mass murders (see boxes: DNA Profiling Identifies September 11 Victims and DNA Identifies Victims of Srebrenica Massacre).

One disadvantage of mtDNA typing is that it cannot distinguish between mtDNA from sib-lings or maternal relatives. It is even possible for two people who are apparently unrelated to share the same mtDNA profile, if they shared a maternal ancestor in the distant past. Also, mtDNA profiles do not provide the same discriminating power as do STR profiles.

Y Chromosome Analysis

Profiling of Y chromosome DNA is used to distinguish multiple male contributors to biological samples. It is useful in sexual assault cases, as most vaginal swabs from rape cases contain a large number of female victim cells and a smaller number of sperm cells. The DNA in X chromosomes does not amplify by Y chromosome-specific PCR, and therefore does not interfere with analysis of Y chromosome loci. Over 100 loci on the Y chromosome are useful as DNA profile loci, including STRs and SNPs.

The Y chromosome is inherited from father to son as a single unpaired chromosome, and it is not present in females. Similar to mtDNA, all the loci on the Y chromosome behave as a single locus that is inherited as a unit. As all males in the paternal line carry the same Y chromosome, this method can also be used to trace family relationships between males, and has been used in human evolution studies.

A complication of Y chromosome profiling is that it cannot distinguish between siblings or other males in the paternal line. In addition, a Y chromosome profile can be shared by those who unknowingly shared a distant male ancestor.

An interesting case in Poland involved Y chromosome analysis to help screen hundreds of men dur-ing a police dragnet for a serial rapist-murderer (see box: Polish Dragnet Apprehends Serial Rapist).

DNA Identifies Victims of Srebrenica Massacre

In July 1995, Serbian troops seized the Bosnian town of Srebrenica. About 25,000 Muslim inhabitants fled—some to the woods and some to the United Nation's (U.N.) compound outside the town. Unfortunately, the compound was full and the gates were locked. The Muslim refugees camped outside the gates, hoping to be protected by U.N. soldiers; however, the Serbian forces arrived unopposed. Over 7,500 men and boys from outside the U.N. compound were shipped to execution sites, killed, and buried in mass graves. Later, the bodies from these graves were dug up and reburied throughout the region in an attempt to conceal evidence. The massacre was the largest mass murder of European civilians since World War II.

In 1996, U.S. President Bill Clinton established the International Commission on Missing Persons (ICMP) to return massacre victims to their families. The goal of ICMP is to identify the approximately 30,000 persons missing in the former Yugoslavia—an effort that will be the world's largest DNA profiling project to identify human remains. By the end of 2002, about 6,000 bodies from the Srebrenica massacre had been exhumed from a number of grave sites and stored in plastic bags in a warehouse near Tuzla. Standard postmortem procedures determine the age, gender, injuries, and general stature of the victims. Clothing is removed, laundered, and displayed for families to identify. However, as identification papers are missing and bodies are severely disfigured and decayed, visual identification is virtually impossible. Only a handful of remains have been identified by standard forensic methods.

The ICMP's DNA profiling will cost approximately $25 million. Outreach programs are collecting thousands of blood samples from relatives of the missing people. In addition, the bones of massacre victims are being cleaned and prepared for analysis. Samples will be sent to four DNA analysis laboratories situated in the former Yugoslavia. The DNA will be extracted from these samples, and relevant regions of nuclear and mitochondrial DNA (mtDNA) will be amplified by PCR. As mitochondrial genomes are often more resistant to degradation than nuclear DNA, mtDNA profiling is expected to provide the most efficient way to identify many of the victims. In addition, there are often surviving maternal relatives who can provide blood samples in order to match the DNA profiles to those of the missing persons. As it

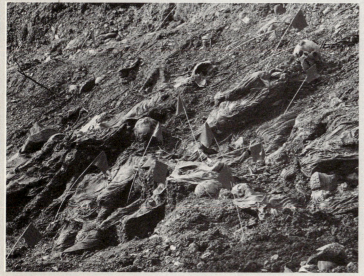

will not be possible to distinguish siblings simply by mitochondrial profiles, additional DNA profiling of STR loci, and Y chromosome markers will be necessary to ascribe names to the thousands of anonymous victims of the Srebrenica massacre.

Identifications are proceeding at a rate of two or three per day. By the end of 2002, over 100 bodies had been identified. However, some remains will never be identified. The names of the missing will be listed at a memorial center in the cemetery outside of Srebrenica.

Mass grave, near Srebrenica.
SOURCE: AP/World Wide Photos

Questions About Interpreting DNA Profiles

WHY ARE DNA PROFILES INTERPRETED IN TERMS OF PROBABILITIES?

A typical DNA forensics case involves comparing the DNA profile from an evidence sample (such as a bloodstain from a murder or a semen sample from a rape) to a profile derived from a suspect (usually from a mouth swab or blood sample).

Polish Dragnet Apprehends Serial Rapist

Over a six-year period, 14 young women between the ages of nine and 26 years were brutally raped near the town of Swinoujscie in northwest Poland. In 2000, one of the rape victims was also murdered. Although the victims described the rapist as tall, athletic, and carrying a handgun, they were unable to identify him because he wore a mask.

Vaginal swabs were obtained from the rape victims, and DNA was analyzed by STR and Y chromosome profiling. The Y chromosome DNA profiles confirmed that all the rapes had been committed by the same man. In one case, a mixture of two profiles was obtained. The victim of this rape reported that she had sexual intercourse with her boyfriend four days prior to the rape. The peak heights of the two superimposed profiles showed that the largest of the peaks for each allele corresponded to the same allele as that of the rapist in the other cases. The STR profiles of 10 autosomal loci also showed mixed alleles, due to a predominance of female cells in the vaginal swabs. By comparing the mixed profiles with the profiles of samples from each of the victims, the profile of the serial rapist was deduced.

In an effort to apprehend the perpetrator of these crimes, the police decided to investigate all young men between the ages of 22 and 38 who lived in the area. Of the 12,000 potential suspects, 714 were interrogated and 421 submitted mouth swabs or blood samples for DNA profiling. Police decided to use Y chromosome profiling in the initial screening to eliminate suspects. One of the 421 Y chromosome profiles (from suspect KW) was identical to the Y chromosome profile obtained from the victims' vaginal swabs. However, when KW's DNA was further analyzed at 10 autosomal STR loci, it did not match perfectly. One of the 10 alleles differed between KW's DNA and the rapist's DNA. This suggested that the rapist was likely to be closely related to KW. Police obtained a mouth swab from KW's brother (TW) and subjected it to both Y chromosome and autosomal STR profiling. Suspect TW's Y chromosome profile and autosomal profile at 19 loci were perfect matches to that of the serial rapist. The chance that this profile would be a random match was estimated to be one in 600 trillion. Several days after the DNA profile results were sent to the public prosecutor, police arrested TW and charged him with committing 14 rapes and one homicide.

SOURCE: A. Dettlaff-Kakol and R. Pawlowski.2002. *First Polish DNA "Manhunt"—An Application of Y-Chromosome STRs*. Int. J. Legal Med. 116:289-291.

There are three possible outcomes of this comparison: the profiles match, the profiles do not match, or the data are inconclusive. If the suspect and evidence samples do not match, it can be concluded that the suspect was not the source of the crime scene sample—therefore, an exclusion. If the DNA profiles from the suspect and evidence samples are indistinguishable, the profiles are said to match. In this case, the samples either came from the same person or came from two different people who simply share the same DNA profiles by chance. In order to present the DNA evidence in such a way as to convey its significance, it is necessary to estimate the probability that the two profiles are a random match.

HOW ARE DNA PROFILE PROBABILITIES CALCULATED AND PRESENTED?

There are several different ways in which match probabilities are calculated. However, the simplest is termed the *profile probability* method. The profile probability is the probability that a person chosen at random from a population would have the same DNA profile as the evidence or suspect samples.

The following is an example of how to calculate a profile probability. This example involves calculating the profile probability at five STR loci as set out in Table 2.

The CSF1PO locus

In this profile of five STR loci, the person exhibited two different-sized alleles at the CSF1PO locus (alleles of 10 and 11 repeats). In the Caucasian American database of 430 alleles (that is, two alleles from each of 215 people sampled), these alleles were observed 108 and 133 times, respectively. Therefore, the frequency of observing these alleles at random in the Caucasian American population

TABLE 2

Locus	DNA Profile				Allele Frequencies from Caucasian American Database		Genotype Frequency in Population	
	Alleles Observed	Times allele observed	Size of Database	Frequency			Formula	Frequency
CSF1PO	10	108	430	$p = 0.25$			$2pq$	0.16
	11	133		$q = 0.31$				
TPOX	8	227	430	$p = 0.53$			p^2	0.28
	8	227		$p = 0.53$				
TH01	6	101	426	$p = 0.24$			$2pq$	0.07
	7	63		$q = 0.15$				
vWA	16	90	426	$p = 0.21$			p^2	0.04
	16	90		$p = 0.21$				
D5S818	13	80	420	$p = 0.19$			$2pq$	0.14
	11	155		$q = 0.37$				

Profile Frequency = 0.00002 (1 in 50,000)

Adapted from: Brenner, C.H., *Forensic Mathematics of DNA Matching*. **http://dna-view.com/profile.htm** and Promega Corporation, Population Data Allele Frequencies.

would be 0.25 (the p frequency) and 0.31 (the q frequency), respectively. The person who contributed this DNA profile can be assumed to have received each of his or her CSF1PO alleles at random from each parent. In other words, the probability of receiving allele 10 from the mother and allele 11 from the father is pq. Similarly, the probability of receiving allele 11 from the mother and allele 10 from the father is also pq. Therefore, the total probability of receiving a 10,11 genotype by chance is $2pq$. In this case, $2pq$ is about 16%. One can see from this example that DNA profiling at one locus is not very discriminating, as about 16% of the population would share this 10,11 DNA profile just by chance. The strength of a profile match, however, increases as one adds more loci to the analysis.

The TPOX locus

This person exhibited two identical TPOX alleles (of 8 repeats) and is therefore homozygous at the TPOX locus. The combined probability of inheriting the eight allele from each parent is $pp = p^2$ and the frequency that one would observe the p^2 genotype in a Caucasian American population would be about 28%. The probability that a person would have a combined TPOX 8,8/CSF1PO 10,11 genotype would be 28% of 16% = about 4%.

The TH01, vWA, and D5S818 loci

The probability calculations for these loci are the same for the remaining loci. By multiplying all the genotype probabilities at the five loci, one obtains an overall profile probability of 0.00002—or a one in 50,000 chance that a person chosen at random from that population would show the same DNA profile.

The method of multiplying all the frequencies of genotypes at each locus is sometimes called the *product rule*. It is the most frequently used method of DNA profile interpretation, and is widely accepted in U.S. courts.

IS A PERSON'S DNA PROFILE UNIQUE?

At present, the FBI uses 13 core STR loci in its profiles. The expected genotype frequency of the most common 13-locus profile would be less than one in 10 billion, and depends slightly upon allele frequencies in different populations. Although these numbers would strongly suggest that two matching profiles came from the same person, they cannot rule out the possibility of a random match.

As one increases the number of loci analyzed in a DNA profile, the probability of a random match in the population becomes smaller. If enough loci were analyzed, one might be certain that the DNA profile is unique. The FBI's policy is that if the match probability is much lower than one in 290 million (U.S. population) then it can be said with reasonable certainty that the DNA profile is unique to one individual.

Several situations exist that modify the profile probability calculations and the interpretation of matching profiles:

- Because they developed from a single fertilized egg, identical twins have identical DNA. Therefore, their DNA profiles will be identical. The frequency of identical twins is about one in every 250 births.

- Because they share parents, siblings often share alleles at any locus. About a quarter of the time, siblings will share both alleles at a particular locus. About half the time, they will share one allele at a locus. Using a DNA profile of 13 core STR loci, the profile probability is about 100,000 times greater if the DNA samples come from siblings than if they come from two unrelated persons. For an example of siblings that matched at a large number of loci, see box: Polish Dragnet Apprehends Serial Rapist.
- A parent and a child will always share one allele at a locus, but they will not usually share two alleles. Other relatives may share a single allele at a locus, but rarely will they share both alleles at a locus.
- The allele frequencies and probability calculations described above are based on the assumption that the population in question is large, with little interrelatedness or inbreeding. For populations that do not meet these assumptions, profile probabilities must be adjusted to reflect certain degrees of interrelatedness.

IF A DEFENDANT'S PROFILE MATCHES THAT OF THE CRIME SCENE SAMPLE, DOES THAT PROVE THE DEFENDANT'S GUILT?

It is important to remember that a match between a crime scene DNA profile and a suspect's profile does not necessarily prove guilt, in the absence of other evidence. As explained in a later section (What Are the Main Problems With Forensic DNA Profiling?), human error or contamination may contribute to a match between a profile from a crime scene sample and a profile from an innocent person. In addition, a suspect's DNA may be introduced to a crime scene before, during, or after the crime for reasons unrelated to the suspect's involvement in the crime. Also, DNA may be introduced to a crime scene by inadvertent or deliberate tampering.

Conversely, a DNA profile exclusion does not necessarily mean innocence. In a rape case, for example, a suspect may not contribute the semen sample, but may have been involved in the crime by restraining the victim. Once again, DNA profiles must always be interpreted in the context of all available evidence.

Questions About the Use of Forensic DNA Profiling

WHAT SORT OF CRIME EVIDENCE IS SUITABLE FOR DNA ANALYSIS?

The sensitivity of PCR-based DNA profiling methods means that any biological material—in theory, even a single cell—can generate a DNA profile. Types of samples include semen from rape cases, bloodspots from murder or assault cases, hairs left behind during robberies, and fingernail scrapings from assaults or murders. Dandruff on hat bands, saliva on cigarette butts, envelopes, stamps, or chewing gum, skin cells on eyeglasses, or even cells from a fingerprint can all generate DNA profiles, as can ear wax, bones, teeth, urine, and feces.

The amounts of biological material necessary to generate a DNA profile can be tiny—as small as the head of a pin or even invisible to the naked eye.

Forensic DNA samples can also be useful when they are decades old and in a partially degraded state. Molecules of DNA are relatively stable to drying, heat, and degradation compared with other types of biological evidence such as enzymes from blood or saliva. In addition, STR and mtDNA loci are small enough that they can be PCR-amplified even if most of the DNA has been degraded into small fragments. Samples of DNA have yielded profiles from the 70-year-old remains of the assassinated Romanov family in Russia, as well as from the prehistoric bones of Kennewick Man in the Pacific Northwest. In theory, DNA profiles can be obtained from samples that are hundreds to thousands of years old.

WHAT ARE THE USES OF FORENSIC DNA PROFILING?

In the United States, the most common forensic use of DNA profiles is in sexual assault cases, as DNA profiles generated from semen on vaginal swabs can provide convincing evidence of a perpetrator. In the United Kingdom, DNA profiles from a wider range of crime scenes, including burglaries, are commonly used. The following list outlines the types of forensic cases that have involved DNA profiling:

- *Convicting the guilty.*
  DNA profiles from rape, murder, burglary, and other crime scenes have been matched with a suspect. Also, DNA profiles from multiple crime scenes have been compared in order to identify common perpetrators.
- *Exonerating the innocent.*
  In the United States, 123 innocent people have been exonerated of their convictions using DNA evidence. Twelve of these were death row inmates, some only days or hours away from execution.
- *Excluding suspects.*
  FBI data show that in sexual assault cases, DNA evidence excludes about 25% of primary suspects prior to trial. This not only allows police forces to redirect investigations at an early stage but also saves resources and the injustice of bringing innocent people to trial.
- *Identifying missing persons.*

DNA profiles obtained from the remains of missing persons have been compared with profiles from relatives in order to establish the identity of body or skeletal remains.

- *Establishing paternity.*
  DNA evidence can help establish parentage. A recent example of DNA profiling in a paternity case is that of Thomas Jefferson, the third president of the United States. The DNA profiling of Y chromosome loci revealed that Jefferson could have fathered children by Sally Hemings, one of his slaves.

- *Identifying military personnel.*
  The military obtains DNA samples from its personnel so as to identify soldiers who may be killed in the line of duty. The bodies of over 500 servicemen and women who died in the Vietnam War have been identified using DNA profiling.

- *Identifying disaster victims.*
  DNA profiling has been employed to identify victims of air crashes such as Swissair Flight 111, which crashed off the coast of Nova Scotia in 1998, and other catastrophes such as the September 11, 2001, terrorist attacks.

- *Identifying victims of mass murders and assassinations.*
  DNA profiling identified the remains of Tsar Nicholas II and members of his family, who were assassinated in Russia in 1918, and also the remains of individuals murdered in Bosnia and Argentina.

- *Identifying protected species (wildlife forensics).*
  DNA samples have been used to determine whether the remains of a particular animal came from an endangered or protected species. Also, DNA profiles have linked an animal's remains with a crime scene or with a suspect.

WHAT ARE THE ADVANTAGES OF DNA EVIDENCE OVER OTHER TYPES OF BIOLOGICAL FORENSIC EVIDENCE?

Forensic DNA evidence has essentially replaced traditional blood typing and saliva testing methods, as it is more sensitive, more informative, and more resilient than older serological methods. Prior to the advent of DNA profiling, combinations of blood types and serum markers could provide match probabilities of about one in several hundred to several thousand. Other biological forensic assays such as microscopic hair analysis have been challenged and will likely be replaced by mtDNA typing in the near future.

HOW RELIABLE IS DNA PROFILE TECHNOLOGY?

In general, the techniques used to generate a DNA profile are highly reliable. Nonetheless, the reliability of DNA profiling can be significantly affected by the methods used to collect, store, and analyze the crime samples, as well as by the interpretation of a profile. For example, during the O.J. Simpson trial, there was relatively little argument with the results of the DNA tests themselves; however, the methods used to collect, store, and handle the crime scene samples shed doubt upon the integrity and origin of the samples used to generate the profiles (see box: The O.J. Simpson Story).

The most persistent problems with PCR-based DNA profiles derive from the presence of contaminants or mixtures in the evidence samples. Contaminants can mix with the evidence

The O.J. Simpson Story

Nicole Brown Simpson and Ronald Goldman were stabbed to death on June 12, 1994, outside Mrs. Simpson's home in Brentwood, California. Actor and ex-football star O.J. Simpson was charged with the murders, and the succeeding trial was one of the most highly publicized trials in American history.

At first it appeared that the forensic DNA evidence against Simpson was overwhelming. The DNA profile from drops of blood leading away from the crime scene were consistent with O.J. Simpson's DNA profile at 5 VNTR loci and 7 PCR DQA1 loci. Also, the DNA profile from blood on a glove found at O.J. Simpson's home was consistent with Mrs. Simpson's profile at 5 VNTR loci and 2 PCR loci, and with Ronald Goldman's profile at 8 VNTR loci and 2 PCR loci. Mrs. Simpson's DNA profile was detected in blood from socks found at the O.J. Simpson home (14 VNTR loci and 7 PCR loci). Expert witnesses testified that such a profile would occur at random in only one of 9.7 billion Caucasians.

Much was made of the DNA profile evidence in this trial. However, in the end, it was the way that the forensic samples had been collected and stored that cast doubt on much of the DNA evidence. Police admitted that they did not wear protective clothing at the crime scene. Photographs showed detectives walking through bloodstains, leaving bloody shoe prints throughout the crime scene as well as outside. This became particularly problematic when it was revealed that detectives who used no protective clothing traveled from the crime scene to O.J. Simpson's residence and potentially could have transferred forensic evidence from one location to another. Defense lawyers showed that a scientist with the Los Angeles Police Department who processed much of the forensic evidence did not change gloves between handling different samples, did not adequately document his blood testing, and failed to follow rules that would ensure against contaminating blood samples. At one point, blood that had been collected from O.J. Simpson was spilled onto plastic gloves and may have contaminated evidence material.

Unimpressed by the prosecution's mountain of DNA evidence and appalled by the apparent sloppiness of police techniques, the jury acquitted O.J. Simpson on two counts of first-degree murder on October 3, 1995.

The O.J. Simpson case was significant in the history of forensic DNA profiling, as it triggered reassessment of police and laboratory procedures for processing crime scene evidence. It also stimulated research on DNA profiling methods and DNA database analysis. The importance of this trial to the development of modern DNA forensics is reflected in the recent donation of the DNA evidence from the O.J. Simpson trial to the Smithsonian Institution.

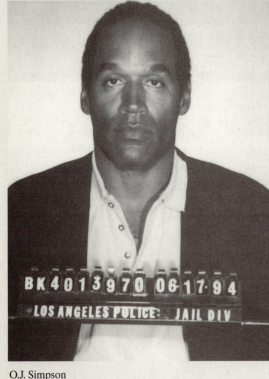

O.J. Simpson

samples before, during, or after their collection, and can come from persons unrelated to the crime, from the investigating officers, or from co-perpetrators of the crime. Current STR technology can often discern the presence of contaminants in a forensic sample, even when these contaminants comprise only 10% of the sample. Contaminants are particularly problematic when there is only a trace amount of evidence material. If the evidence sample contains biological material from two or more people, there will be three or more bands at each STR locus. If the mixture contains STR loci with some identical alleles, the peaks for these alleles will be twice as high. By examining more than one sample from the crime scene, it is often possible to discriminate between alleles in a mixture. Nonetheless, the presence of contaminants and mixtures must be taken into account during presentation of DNA evidence, and may affect the interpretations of profiles.

The National Research Council (NRC) recommends that forensic laboratories in the United States be accredited for doing DNA testing so as to standardize methods and quality. To date, not all private laboratories or police department forensic laboratories are accredited. The NRC also recommends that laboratories routinely use positive and negative controls and take periodic proficiency tests. Another recommendation is that forensic samples be divided into two or more portions so that samples can be retested at a later date. As yet, these recommendations have not been made mandatory for all DNA analysis facilities.

WHAT ARE THE MAIN PROBLEMS WITH FORENSIC DNA PROFILING?

Although DNA profiling methods are highly sensitive and accurate, limitations exist. Most forensic cases do not involve biological evidence, and in those that do, the evidence may not be informative. Evidence may be degraded and yield no profile or may give partial profiles that are not informative.

Not all cases that could benefit by DNA evidence are able to do so. In the United States, about 20% of all rape samples that are collected are not processed. In New York City, the backlog of untested rape samples numbers about 16,000. Nationwide, more than 500,000 DNA samples from convicted prisoners are backlogged and untested, and about 1 million violent offenders who are on supervised release remain untested.

As described in the answer to the previous question, contamination can be a serious complication in the interpretation of a DNA profile. Over the last decade, police have become better trained in collecting crime scene evidence and in documenting the chain of custody of evidence samples. However, the possibility of contamination, either inadvertently or planted, needs to be considered. It might be necessary to obtain profiles from family members or crime scene officers in order to eliminate contaminating bands in a DNA profile. In rape cases, it might be necessary to obtain a DNA sample from anyone having consensual intercourse with the victim within four days prior to the assault, as DNA profiles may be mixed.

One of the most serious complications is human error, either innocent or intentional. An example of human error is illustrated by the Sotolusson case (see box: The Sotolusson Story). Although human error is impossible to eliminate, consideration of all the evidence in a case may pinpoint those instances where accidental or intentional errors have occurred.

The Sotolusson Story

In 2001, Lazaro Sotolusson was arrested for a technical immigration violation in Las Vegas, Nevada. While in prison, his cellmate accused him of rape. Samples of DNA were taken from both inmates, and the forensics laboratory ran the profiles through the Nevada State DNA database. Sotolusson's DNA profile matched profiles from two unsolved rapes in 1998 and 1999, and he was arrested for sexual assault and first-degree kidnapping. Experts stated that the chance of a random match to Sotolusson's profile was about 1 in 600 billion—convincing evidence that could convict him of these rapes. In addition, during a preliminary hearing, one of the rape victims identified Sotolusson as the perpetrator.

A year later, just before the trial, Sotolusson's lawyer hired an independent DNA expert who discovered that Sotolusson's name had been accidentally switched with the name of his cellmate prior to entering the DNA data into the database. The forensics laboratory admitted its mistake, and all sexual assault charges against Sotolusson were dismissed. Sotolusson had spent a year in prison for two crimes that he did not commit. Police are now investigating Sotolusson's former prison cellmate as a suspect in the two rapes.

This case demonstrates how easily human error, in combination with the persuasiveness of DNA profiling, can lead to the arrest of an innocent person.

Questions About the Use, Collection, and Storage of DNA Profiles

HOW MANY PROFILES ARE IN THE CODIS DATABANKS?

At the end of 2002, there were over 1 million profiles entered into the Convicted Offender database and over 44,000 profiles in the Forensic Evidence database. Over 5 million DNA profiles will be entered into CODIS within the next five years. All but three U.S. states have submitted profiles to the CODIS national database. The CODIS system has contributed to about 6,400 criminal investigations and has yielded over 6,000 matches between submitted profiles.

WHOSE DNA PROFILES SHOULD BE INCLUDED IN DNA PROFILE DATABASES?

Although DNA profile databases are rapidly proving to be valuable aids in criminal investigations, their use raises some serious ethical and legal questions concerning the collection and storage of DNA evidence as well as the intended uses of the databases.

Laws and standards for DNA profile collection vary dramatically both within the United States and internationally. In the United Kingdom, everyone arrested for any offense that carries a prison term is obliged to provide a DNA sample. These samples and the profiles generated from them can be retained by police and entered into the U.K.'s national DNA databank. In addition, the United Kingdom permits police to conduct mass screenings (dragnets) to gather profiles from large numbers of people in a given area in attempts to find a suspect. There have been 120 such dragnets in England and Wales. In the United States, rules governing DNA sample collection and database entry form a state-by-state patchwork. The CODIS rules limit DNA profiles to those from convicted offenders. However, state-based databases do not necessarily follow these same rules. For example, some states permit the taking of a suspect's DNA sample at the time of arrest. One state (Ohio) is reported to retain all profiles regardless of whether the suspect is convicted. Other states restrict sample collection to convicted offenders only, or to offenders convicted of specific violent crimes. Some states allow juveniles to be DNA profiled and others do not. There have even been cases where DNA dragnets were carried out, and the profiles and samples retained.

The intended uses of DNA profile databanks also vary. Some states allow databanks to be used for any criminal investigation, but others limit searches to sex-related or violent crimes. The CODIS rules allow searching the databases for any criminal investigation.

In the United States, considerable interest exists in expanding DNA database entries to all arrestees. Although there are clear advantages, such as the ability of police to exclude suspects early in an investigation and to find perpetrators through database searches, many people are alarmed at this prospect and demand that safeguards be in place. Most believe that profiles and samples must be expunged from the system if the suspect is not charged, or if a suspect is found not guilty. Many critics question the expansion of DNA databases, based on the Fourth Amendment, which protects citizens against unreasonable search and seizure. So far, legal challenges to DNA sample collection and database entry have been unsuccessful. Some people question DNA databanks on the basis of social inequality. Because some groups, such as African Americans, are overrepresented in convictions, they may also be overrepresented in DNA databanks. Some critics of the present system of DNA databanking argue that universal DNA profiling of all citizens would be a fairer policy than profiling only certain individuals. Such an idea raises even more questions about how personal privacy would be safeguarded for profiles held by police and governments.

AFTER DNA PROFILING AND ELECTRONIC STORAGE OF THE PROFILE, SHOULD THE TISSUE SAMPLE BE RETAINED OR DESTROYED?

Another contentious question is that of tissue sample retention. Forensic experts have argued that tissue samples should be retained in case the currently used 13-core STR loci system becomes superseded by a newer and more efficient system, such as the emerging SNP and mtDNA technologies. Also, retention of the original samples would allow retesting in the event of a suspected technical error. Others argue that the original samples should be destroyed after DNA profiles are generated so as to protect citizens from present and future unauthorized use of the samples. Currently, state laws vary as to the retention of samples and DNA profiles from people found innocent or those who have been wrongly convicted.

CAN PERSONAL OR MEDICAL INFORMATION BE OBTAINED FROM DNA PROFILES?

One of the concerns about DNA databases is that they may allow authorities to violate a person's genetic privacy and obtain information about a person's disease susceptibility, race, physical features, or parentage. Another concern is that databases could be used for genetic research without the consent of those in the database. At present, the loci used for DNA profiling are not known to be associated with any physical or behavioral traits. However, in the future it may be possible to link DNA profile information with physical characteristics that would help police identify a suspect.

Also, DNA databases have the potential to point toward close relatives of a suspect. For example, a crime scene DNA profile may partially match that of a convicted offender whose profile is located in the offender database. A partial match, although excluding the offender, might suggest that a sibling or other close relative of that offender may match the profile (see box: Polish Dragnet Apprehends Serial Rapist). It is a matter of debate whether police should have the right to obtain profiles from relatives under these circumstances, without any other probable cause for obtaining the information. States differ in their rules about the admissibility of pursuing offender's relatives based on partial DNA matches.

Questions About DNA Profiling and the Criminal Justice System

HOW CAN DNA EVIDENCE EXONERATE THOSE WHO ARE WRONGLY CONVICTED?

Since 1992, over 120 convicted prisoners, including 12 on death row, have been exonerated based on DNA evidence. Most of these exonerations were for cases tried prior to 1994, when DNA profiling was either not available or required large amounts of DNA for VNTR analysis. Now that modern DNA profiling methods can generate information on small quantities of DNA that are degraded and even decades old, convictions are being challenged and some are being overturned. In over a dozen cases, DNA evidence not only exonerated an innocent inmate, but also led to the identification of the perpetrator through DNA database searches.

Some people find the rising number of post-conviction exonerations disturbing, not only because of the injustice of incarcerating and perhaps executing innocent people, but also because the perpetrator of these crimes may remain free to commit more offences. In January 2003, Illinois Governor George Ryan commuted all death sentences to life in prison without parole, after learning that the state had executed 12 death row prisoners, but exonerated 13, some based on DNA evidence. Governor Ryan was concerned that innocent people could have been executed in the absence of post-conviction evidence disproving their guilt.

It is difficult to estimate how many inmates could be exonerated if DNA testing was available to illuminate their cases. The majority of criminal cases do not involve biological evidence, and of those that do, the evidence may be destroyed or lost over the years. The Innocence Project, a nonprofit legal clinic at the Benjamin N. Cardozo School of Law in New York, has taken on 123 cases in which DNA evidence led to post-conviction exonerations. Thousands more have requested assistance, but in about 75% of cases, the biological evidence cannot be located. Presumably the number of exonerations would increase if DNA samples were available. For examples of post-conviction exonerations based upon DNA profiling, see boxes: The Marvin Anderson Story, and The Earl Washington Story.

Despite the power of post-conviction DNA testing to exonerate the innocent and identify the guilty, obstacles prevent its routine use or effectiveness. For example, current U.S. laws limit the time during which convicted people can introduce new evidence, usually less than two or three years following conviction. In some instances, exonerations have been delayed or prevented when the prosecution introduced a new theory about the case that was not part of the original trial. In addition, many suspects and convicts are indigent and cannot afford the costs of DNA testing or adequate legal counsel to challenge their arrests or convictions.

The Marvin Anderson Story

In July 1982, a young white woman in Ashland, Virginia, was raped by a black man who had approached her on a bicycle. The rapist threatened her with a gun, then beat, raped, and sodomized her. He then bragged to her that he "had a white girl."

After the victim reported the crime, the police focused on Marvin Anderson as a suspect, as he was the only black man in the area that the police knew who had a white girl friend. Anderson had no criminal record, so police obtained a photo from Anderson's employer, using it in a photo lineup. From the photo lineup, the victim picked Anderson as the rapist. In the subsequent suspect lineup, the victim also picked out Anderson. He was the only person in the suspect lineup whose photo was also in the photo lineup. Serological analyses of rape samples were not informative.

Although Anderson was charged with the crime, members of the community suspected that the real rapist was probably another man named John Otis Lincoln. Lincoln had stolen a bicycle less than an hour before the rape, and the bicycle was identified by the owner. Anderson requested that both the bicycle's owner and Lincoln himself testify at the trial, however, his legal counsel refused. On December 14, 1982, an all-white jury convicted Marvin Anderson of robbery, forcible sodomy, abduction, and two counts of rape. He was sentenced to 210 years in the Virginia State Penitentiary.

Six years later, John Otis Lincoln admitted that he had committed the crime. However, the judge that had presided over Anderson's trial refused to accept Lincoln's confession. Anderson's case was taken up by civil rights groups, church leaders, and Virginia politicians. However, Governor Wilder denied their request for clemency in 1993. Anderson attempted to prove his innocence by demanding DNA analysis of the rape samples. Authorities informed his lawyers that the rape samples had been destroyed.

In 1994, Marvin Anderson's case was accepted by the Innocence Project. In 2001, Virginia's Division of Forensic Science informed the Innocence Project that the rape samples had been found—taped into the laboratory notebook of the forensic scientist who had done the conventional serology tests in 1982. This mistake by the forensics lab had saved the vaginal swabs from being destroyed.

On December 6, 2001, partial DNA profiles generated from the old rape evidence excluded Marvin Anderson as the perpetrator of the crimes. The DNA profile was run through Virginia's offender DNA database, and it matched the profiles of two inmates. One of these profiles is reported to be from John Otis Lincoln.

Marvin Anderson had spent 15 years in prison and four years on parole for a crime he did not commit. He became the 99th person in the United States to be exonerated based on post-conviction DNA profiling.

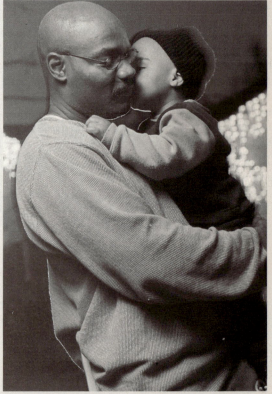

Marvin Anderson, with his son, after his exoneration in December 2001.
SOURCE: *New York Times* Pictures

The Earl Washington Story

In June 1982, a 19-year-old white woman, Rebecca Williams, was raped and murdered in her Culpeper, Virginia, apartment. Before she died, she told police that she had been assaulted by a black man.

A year later, Earl Washington, a 22-year-old farmhand with an IQ of 69, was arrested for an alleged burglary and malicious wounding. Police questioned Washington for two days, during which time he confessed to five different crimes, including the rape and murder of Rebecca Williams. Four of the confessions were dismissed when witnesses stated that Washington was not the perpetrator. However, the murder confession remained and he was charged. Washington's murder confession was taken by a Virginia state trooper who asked, "Did you kill the woman in Culpeper?" and "Did you stab the woman in Culpeper?" Washington replied, "Yes, sir." However, when asked for details of the murder, he was not able to supply them. He did not know the race or height of the victim, how the crime was committed, or the location of the apartment.

The confession was the only evidence linking Earl Washington to the rape and murder of Rebecca Williams. Serological tests on blood and semen stains were inconclusive. Psychological tests showed that Washington politely agreed with any authority figure in order to gain approval and to compensate for his mental disabilities. Washington's legal defense did not bring out the results of the psychological tests, the inconsistencies in his confession, the weaknesses in the prosecution's case, or even argue against the sentence.

Earl Washington's trial lasted three days. On January 20, 1984, he was convicted of murder and sentenced to death.

Nine days before he was to be executed, lawyers from a New York firm obtained a stay of execution and later appealed Washington's conviction. Although the court agreed that Washington had been denied his constitutional right to effective counsel, his confession was still accepted and his conviction upheld.

In 1993, Earl Washington's lawyers asked Virginia Governor Wilder to grant Washington a pardon. The governor requested DNA tests before making a decision. Results showed that semen on the vaginal swab could not have come from Washington. At this point, a new prosecution theory emerged: Earl Washington, along with someone else who contributed the DNA in the semen stain, was responsible for the crime. Although there was no evidence that two people were involved in the crime, the theory gained credence. On the last day of Governor Wilder's term, Washington and his counsel were given two hours to accept commutation of the death sentence to life imprisonment without parole. They accepted.

Earl Washington remained in prison for another six years before his lawyers were able to persuade Governor Gilmore to do more DNA testing. On October 2, 2000, the governor announced that the STR (short tandem repeat) DNA profiles from the crime scene evidence excluded Earl Washington and granted his absolute pardon. Finally, on February 12, 2001, Earl Washington was released from prison into parole supervision, 17 years after his wrongful murder conviction.

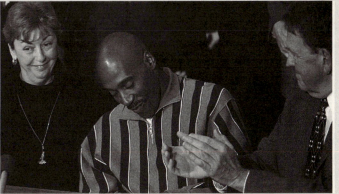

Earl Washington with his lawyers, Marie Deans and Robert T. Hall, after his exoneration from rape charges on February 12, 2001, in Virginia Beach, Virginia.
SOURCE: AP/World Wide Photos

WHY ARE INNOCENT PEOPLE CONVICTED OF VIOLENT CRIMES AND THEN EXONERATED?

The Innocence Project and the U.S. Department of Justice have studied DNA-based exonerations and have identified a number of common features. The most common cause of wrongful conviction is mistaken eyewitness testimony. It has been shown that eyewitness testimony is the least dependable, but most persuasive, evidence in a court case. Memory is extremely plastic and unreliable even when the victim attempts to carefully remember the perpetrator. Time, stress, and confusion can lead to a false identification. In addition, eyewitnesses can be influenced by the composition of police lineups. If the perpetrator is not present in the lineup, victims tend to pick the person who best fits their memory, and this identification becomes fixed in their minds. Also, police can sometimes unwittingly lead the victim to choose the suspect that they favor.

Another surprising cause of wrongful convictions is false confession. About 20% of DNA exonerations have occurred in cases where defendants confessed to a crime they did not commit. Police interrogation techniques and the mental incapacity of the suspect are important factors in false confessions. The cases of Earl Washington (see box: The Earl Washington Story) and Colin Pitchfork (see box: The Colin Pitchfork Story) illustrate how a false confession can lead to a wrongful conviction.

About half of DNA-based exonerations involve misconduct of prosecutors or police—for example, by using forced confessions or manufactured evidence. About one-third involve incompetent or inadequate defense counsel, usually when the defendant was indigent and relied on public defenders with inadequate resources or training. In 25 of the first 82 exonerations based on DNA evidence, the court was swayed by fraudulent or "junk" science. Expert witnesses lied about, misinterpreted, exaggerated, or suppressed scientific test results (see Ray Krone's story in the Introduction). For further information about the causes and remedies of wrongful convictions, see the Innocence Project's Web site: (www.innocenceproject.org).

IS IT POSSIBLE FOR AN INNOCENT PERSON TO BE CONVICTED BASED ON DNA EVIDENCE?

So far, there appear to be no cases in which a PCR-based DNA profile led to a wrongful conviction; however, it is feasible that it could happen. Current techniques in DNA profiling are extremely sensitive, with the capacity to generate a profile from only a few cells. It is possible for an innocent person's DNA to be found at a crime scene, either from directly depositing cells at the scene, or from having the cells introduced indirectly by a third person or object. If the innocent person's DNA masks or substitutes for the DNA of the real perpetrator in one or more crime scene samples, it is possible that his or her profile could contribute to a conviction. It is standard practice to obtain elimination samples from family members and investigators who have access to a crime scene, or from consensual sexual partners in a rape case; however, innocent people may contribute material to a crime scene and not be eliminated in this way. It would be relatively simple to plant DNA evidence at a crime scene, as very little material would be required to generate an incriminating profile. Crime scene evidence is not always in good condition, leading to partial profiles that detect only a few loci. It is possible for the profile of an innocent person whose DNA is in a DNA databank to match a partial profile from the crime scene. Close relatives of perpetrators, conceivably even identical twins, could also be incriminated based on partial profiles. Given the fallibility of other types of evidence such as eyewitness identification, and the possibility of false confessions and inadequate defense counsel, it is not impossible for modern DNA profiling to contribute to a wrongful conviction. In light of these possibilities, it is important to remember that the relevance of DNA profiling must be assessed in the context of all evidence in a case.

HOW IS DNA EVIDENCE CHANGING THE U.S. CRIMINAL JUSTICE SYSTEM?

Over the last decade, forensic DNA profiling has significantly altered the operation of the criminal justice system. Old cases are being reexamined, leading to exonerations of innocent prisoners and identification of perpetrators from searches of databases. By using DNA profiling early in an investigation, police are able to exclude innocent suspects, saving both time and effort in locating the real perpetrator. In the future, DNA profiling will undoubtedly reduce the number of wrongful convictions, particularly in sexual assault cases where DNA evidence has the power to convincingly identify a perpetrator.

The ever increasing number of exonerations of wrongfully convicted prisoners, based on re-examination of DNA evidence, has pointed out significant problems with many aspects of the criminal justice system. Police techniques that lead to false confessions and faulty eyewitness identifications have been seriously examined and reforms outlined. Police are being trained in the collection, storage, and chain of custody of forensic evidence, to avoid the types of challenges that arose in cases such as the O.J. Simpson trial. There is now pressure to accredit and review the operations of forensic laboratories, as well as to ensure that such facilities are independent of law enforcement agencies, as is the case in the United Kingdom and Canada. Evidence from DNA samples also challenges many traditional and controversial forensic methods. For example, methods such as microscopic hair examination will likely be replaced by more accurate STR and mtDNA testing.

Perhaps the most profound effect of DNA forensics has been its convincing proof that the system sends innocent people to death row. This revelation has triggered legislative efforts to remedy the situation. In 2002, the Innocence Protection Act was introduced in the U.S. House of Representatives. This legislation would grant convicted prisoners the right to have DNA testing done if the test has the potential to establish innocence. It also outlines measures to ensure that evidence is preserved, and that testing will be paid for by the state in cases of indigence. The legislation would also establish standards for legal representation in capital cases, would set minimum levels of compensation for years of wrongful incarceration, and would ensure that prisoners are not executed while their cases are being heard by the U.S. Supreme Court. The Innocence Protection Act is expected to be passed in 2003.

In the future, DNA profiling will continue to alter criminal justice systems around the world. In order to protect society and individuals from potential abuses, the power of this technology must be tempered by safeguards. Governments must devise rules dealing with DNA databanking, the taking and storing of DNA samples, and the accreditation of DNA analysis laboratories. Police, lawyers, judges, and the public must be informed about the pros and cons of forensic DNA profiling so as to evaluate it and question it intelligently. In addition, sufficient funding must be allocated to ensure that all suspects and convicted persons have full and impartial access to this powerful new technology.

REFERENCES AND RESOURCES

PUBLICATIONS

National Institute of Justice. 2000. *The Future of Forensic DNA Testing: Predictions of the Research and Development Working Group*. (**http://www.ncjrs.org/pdffiles1/nij/183697.pdf**)

National Institute of Justice, National Commission on the Future of DNA Evidence. 2002. *Using DNA to Solve Cold Cases*. (**http://www.ncjrs.org/pdffiles1/nij/194197.pdf**)

National Research Council, Commission of DNA Forensic Science: An Update. 1996. *The Evaluation of Forensic DNA Evidence*. National Academy Press. (**http://search.nap.edu/readingroom/books/DNA/**)

Weedn, V.W. and Hicks, J.W. 1998. *The Unrealized Potential of DNA Testing*. National Institute of Justice, U.S. Department of Justice. (**http://www.ncjrs.org/pdffiles/170596.pdf**)

Connors, E. et al. 1996. *Convicted by Juries, Exonerated by Science: Case Studies in the Use of DNA Evidence to Establish Innocence After Trial*. National Institute of Justice, U.S. Department of Justice. (**http://www.ncjrs.org/pdffiles/dnaevid.pdf**)

Reilly, P. 2001. *Legal and Public Policy Issues in DNA Forensics*. *Nature Reviews Genetics* 2:313–317.

Gill, P. 2002. *Role of Short Tandem Repeat DNA in Forensic Casework in the UK—Past, Present and Future Perspectives*. *BioTechniques* 32:366–385.

Hand, L. 2002. *SNP Technology Focuses on Terror Victims' IDs*. *The Scientist* 16:20.

Ruitberg, C.M. et al. 2001. *STRBase: A Short Tandem Repeat DNA Database for the Human Identity Testing Community*. *Nucleic Acids Res* 29:320–322.

Bunk, S. 2000. *Forensics Fights Crimes Against Wildlife: DNA Technologies Can Nab a Killer, Even When the Victim Is a Moose or Bear*. *The Scientist* 14:24.

Robb, N. 1999. *229 People, 15,000 Body Parts: Pathologists Help Solve Swissair 111's Grisly Puzzles*. *Can Med Assoc J* 160:241–243.

Miller, K.A. 2002. *Identifying Those Remembered: New Technologies Promise to Speed DNA Identification at Disaster Sites and in Criminal Investigations*. *The Scientist* 16:40.

Lipton, E. and Glanz, J. 2002. *A Nation Challenged: Forensics; DNA Science Pushed to the Limit in Identifying the Dead of Sept. 11*. *The New York Times*, April 22, 2002.

Puit, G. *DNA Evidence: Officials Admit Error, Dismiss Case*. *Las Vegas Review–Journal*, April 18, 2002. (**http://www.forensicdna.com/DNAerror.htm**)

Carey, L. and Mitnik, L. 2002. *Trends in DNA Forensic Analysis*. *Electrophoresis* 23:1386–1397.

Williamson, R. and Duncan, R. 2002. *DNA Testing for All*. *Nature* 418:585–586.

WEB SITES

The Innocence Project **http://www.innocenceproject.org**

Forensic mathematics of DNA matching, by Charles H. Brenner, Ph.D. **http://dna-view.com/profile.htm**

DNA Technology links **http://www.law-forensic.com/dnalinks.htm**

True Crimes Criminal Investigations—DNA & Forensic Science **http://www.karisable.com/crdna1.htm**

STRBase: short tandem repeat DNA internet database **http://www.cstl.nist.gov/biotech/strbase/**

"The Case for Innocence: Why do inmates remain in prison despite DNA evidence which exonerates them with near certainty?" PBS Frontline program, 2000. **http://www.pbs.org/wgbh/pages/frontline/shows/case/**

"What Jennifer Saw: Ronald Cotton's wrongful conviction" PBS Frontline program, 1998. **http://www.pbs.org/wgbh/pages/frontline/shows/dna/cotton**

Kennewick Man DNA testing **http://www.cr.nps.gov/aad/kennewick/**

Romanovs find closure in DNA **http://users.rcn.com/web-czar/dna.htm**

The Innocence Protection Act of 2001 (Introduced in the U.S. House of Representatives) **http://thomas.loc.gov/cgi-bin/query/z?c107:H.R.912:**

How DNA technology is reshaping judicial process and outcome Co-sponsored by CSIS and the Whitehead Institute for Biomedical Research, May 2001. **http://www.csis.org/tech/Biotech/nbpp/Seminar2Brief.htm**

DNA Forensics. Human Genome Project Information **http://www.ornl.gov/hgmis/elsi/forensics.html**

Forensic Bioinformatics, Inc., a private company that provides independent reviews of forensic DNA evidence. **http://www.bioforensics.com**